BACK THERAPY

THE HEALING TOUCH

Proven Strategies To Relieve and Reverse Back Problems

Haven Davidson

Copyright © 2020 Haven Davidson

All Rights Reserved

Copyright 2020 By Haven Davidson - All rights reserved.

The following book is produced below with the goal of providing information that is as accurate and reliable as possible. Regardless, purchasing this eBook can be seen as consent to the fact that both the publisher and the author of this book are in no way experts on the topics discussed within and that any recommendations or suggestions that are made herein are for entertainment purposes only. Professionals should be consulted as needed prior to undertaking any of the action endorsed herein.

This declaration is deemed fair and valid by both the American Bar Association and the Committee of Publishers Association and is legally binding throughout the United States.

Furthermore, the transmission, duplication or reproduction of any of the following work including specific information will be considered an illegal act irrespective of if it is done electronically or in print. This extends to creating a secondary or tertiary copy of the work or a recorded copy and is only allowed with express written consent from the Publisher. All additional right reserved.

The information in the following pages is broadly considered to be a truthful and accurate account of facts and as such any inattention, use or misuse of the information in question by the reader will render any resulting actions solely under their purview. There are no scenarios in which the publisher or the original author of this work can be in any fashion deemed liable for any hardship or damages that may befall them after undertaking information described herein.

Additionally, the information in the following pages is intended only for informational purposes and should thus be thought of as universal. As befitting its nature, it is presented without assurance regarding its prolonged validity or interim quality. Trademarks that are mentioned are done without written consent and can in no way be considered an endorsement from the trademark holder.

Table of Contents

PART I 8
Chapter 2: Causes of Back Pain 15
Chapter 3: 21
All About TMS in the Mind and Body 21
Chapter 4: Posture 26
Chapter 5: 31
Improper Treatment and Diagnosis 31
Chapter 6: Treating Back Pain 35
Chapter 7: Traditional Healing Methods 42
Chapter 8: 55
Exercises to Alleviate Symptoms 55
Chapter 9: In Case of Emergency 69
PART II 73
Chapter 1: How to Choose the Right Number of Repetitions 74
Chapter 2: How to Breathe During Exercises 78
Chapter 3: Machines or Free Weights? 81
Chapter 4: Putting it all together. How to program a training cycle ... 85
Chapter 1: Setting Yourself Up For Success 92
   How Your Diet Affects Your Results 92
   Warm Up Before Working Out 92
   Who These Workouts Are Best-Suited For 94
   Benefits of Bodyweight Workouts 94
   Creating a Workout Environment 96
   Summary and Key Points 97
Chapter 2: Types of Bodyweight Workouts 98
   Summary and Key Points 105
Chapter 3: Planning a Workout Routine That Works For You 106
   What to Include In Your Plan 106
   How to Stay Dedicated When Your Resolve Falters 107
   Sample 7-day Routine 109
   Summary and Key Points 112
Chapter 4: How to Make the Most Out of Your Bodyweight Workouts 113
   High-Intensity Interval Training 113
   Progress Can Be Small, But Any Progress is Significant 113
   Technology Can Help Us Keep More Accurate Records 114
   Stretching for Injury Prevention Should Be a Priority 114
   Key Summary Points 114
Taking 5-15 minutes to stretch after a workout will ease soreness for your workouts in the following days, and will help prevent your muscles from getting injured. 115
Conclusion 116

PART I

Introduction

Back pain is something that affects a large majority of the population. In fact, it is estimated that as much as 10% of the population suffers from pain in their back for a number of different reasons.

Back, neck and shoulder pain can have an incredibly negative effect on how we live our lives. It can affect everything from how we sleep to how we participate in daily activities, and even our overall moods. When someone struggles with chronic back, neck, or shoulder pain, they are a lot less likely to be able to participate in regular daily activities and maintain elevated moods. Back pain can be a great source of stress and discomfort, leading to many difficult emotions that result as a backlash of not being able to participate comfortably in mandatory and enjoyable every day activities.

If you are someone who suffers with chronic back, neck, and/or shoulder pain, rest assured you are not alone. There are many people in the world who suffer also. Furthermore, there are many opportunities for you to take action on solutions that truly work. *"Standing Upright*: The Proven 30 Day Solution to Neck, Back and Shoulder Pain" is designed for people who are looking for solutions for their back problems. These solutions do not revolve around medications or other Western medicines, but rather around finding the true ailment and the natural and proven solution to help you relieve your back pain. While there may be some instances where medicines are necessary, we are all for finding the true problem and healing it so that you are free of pain, instead of simply numbing out the symptoms.

If you have been searching for solutions to your back, neck or shoulder pains, then you have come to the right place. This book is filled with proven solutions that will have you feeling significantly better in as little as thirty days. These solutions are gathered from highly skilled doctors from all around the world who specialize in helping people who suffer with chronic back pain find permanent solutions for their problems. I can guarantee that you will find a solution for your own back pain within' this book. If you are ready to start living pain free and enjoying your life again, read on!

Chapter 1: Living with Back Pain

Living with back pain can be incredibly difficult. Those who struggle with back pain know that this type of pain can negatively affect virtually every area of your life. From completing every day activities, to simply trying to enjoy life, back pain can make everything a lot more difficult. The following will help you get insight as to how your life is affected when you live with back pain.

Daily Tasks

When you live with back pain, even simple daily tasks can be negatively affected. There are only three ways a person can be oriented: laying down, sitting, or standing. When you have back, neck, or shoulder pain, all three of these orientations can be negatively affected, leaving you to feel like there is nothing you can do to be pain free.

Sleeping can be one of the hardest parts of having back pain. When you sleep, you may find some comfortable positions that reduce the amount of pain you feel, but actually getting comfortable and getting a quality night's sleep can be nearly impossible.

If you work in a job that requires you to sit or stand for long periods of time, it can be difficult to accomplish this job. Maintaining your position and staying in it for a long period of time can worsen your pain, making it even harder to get your job done.

When it comes to doing everyday tasks such as grocery shopping, dressing, preparing meals, driving, walking, or otherwise living your life, it can be just as difficult to get these done. Back pain touches literally every part of your life, making almost everything you do just that much more difficult. There is nearly no part of your life that goes untouched when you experience chronic back, neck, or shoulder pain for any length of time.

Independence

People with chronic back pain don't always have the opportunity to be entirely independent. Since completing everyday tasks can be so difficult, they may find themselves relying on others to help them. If they don't, they may find themselves in a position where they take on a task that worsens their pain, making everything that much more difficult for themselves in the long run.

Relying on others to help you accomplish everyday tasks can be difficult. Not only are you unable to do them yourself, but you also have to wait for others to be available to help you. Some people report this to be very embarrassing, sometimes even causing them to feel like a burden on relatives or friends because they require so much help to get certain things done. Losing your independence to chronic back pain, no matter what your age, can be difficult.

Quality of Life

In general, people with chronic back pain don't experience the quality of life they could if they were feeling healthy and free of pain. The emotional burdens that can come with being in chronic pain are heavy, often leading to many people feeling depressive episodes. They may also experience anxiety, anger, stress, and other uncomfortable emotions.

When you deal with chronic back pain, every part of your life is touched from your ability to accomplish physical tasks, to even your mental endurance. There is an extensive number of symptoms related to chronic back pain that aren't just the back pain itself. Dealing with these symptoms can be difficult, and can greatly decrease the quality of life for those struggling with their symptoms of chronic back pain.

Overall, living with chronic back pain can have a significantly negative impact on your life. That is why you are likely seeking the opportunity to find the root of the cause and heal yourself from these struggles. This book will help you change your story so that you are no longer losing the quality of your life, your independence, and your comfort to back, neck or shoulder pain.

Chapter 2: Causes of Back Pain

Before you can begin to treat your back pain, you need to understand why you have it in the first place. Many modern treatments simply cover up the symptoms. We will discuss these treatments more, later. If you want true relief from your pain, however, you need to understand that this comes from actually finding the root of the problem and healing it. It does not come by simply hiding the symptoms with the use of pain medicines.

There are many reasons why people suffer from back pain, but there are some very common ones that are experienced by a large majority of the population. The following conditions will explain how you may have acquired your back pain so that you can identify the root cause and then find the perfect solution to your pains.

Posture

Posture is the leading cause for chronic back pain experienced by those with no actual health conditions. Many people in modern society do not pay attention to carrying a proper posture, and this can result in having a sore back, neck, and shoulders, as well as pain in your muscles and joints overall. If you have poor posture and are experiencing these symptoms, it is likely that your posture is the root of your back pain. In order to heal your back pain, you would need to adjust your posture and practice exercises that will heal your posture-related symptoms.

Weak Muscles

Many people don't realize that having a weak core is actually a large cause for having back pain, particularly in the lower back. When your abdominal muscles are strong, you use them when you are lifting or carrying things. When they are not, that burden is put onto your back and your spine. This results in severe lower back pain, which can sometimes spread up into the shoulders and neck if it is left for too long. If you are struggling with back pain as a result of weak muscles, the best course of action would be to start working on building up your core muscles and teaching them to relieve your back of the burden when it comes to carrying weight.

Genetics

Some people are born with genetic conditions that are responsible for their lower back pain. Conditions such as Lumbar Disc Degeneration, Rheumatic Arthritis, and other conditions can be inherited and can be responsible for your lower back pain. If you have anyone in your family who has had a condition that has resulted in them having lower back pain, or back pain in general, the best course of action is to communicate with your doctor and press for answers on what the root cause is. If they do diagnose you with a condition that may be related to your back pain and that was inherited, then you have a solid answer that you can use to help you discover ways to relieve your pain.

Structural Abnormalities

Structural abnormalities can be genetic, or they can be the result of poor posture. People who have genetic structural abnormalities may have conditions such as scoliosis that alter the natural shape of the spine and result in severe pain in the back. Those with poor posture for long periods of time may cause for their back to be put out of position and result in "taught" structural abnormalities. Structural abnormalities have a variety of treatments, depending on the specific cause. Conditions like scoliosis, for example, may be alleviated using spinal surgery. For those who have spinal structure abnormalities as a result of posture, however, correcting the posture and considering chiropractic care can greatly help eliminate the pain felt in the back and shoulders.

Weight, Age, Height

Factors such as your weight, age and height can all contribute to whether or not you will feel back, neck, or shoulder pain. For example, those who are heavier set may find that they have more back pain as a result of their back carrying the stress of more weight on the front of them. Those who are taller may also feel more back, shoulder and neck pain as a result of gravity pulling down on them and creating stress in their muscles. Older people tend to be weaker, which results in weakened muscles and therefore increased likelihood of back pain. If you have any combination of these three, then you are a prime candidate for back, neck, and shoulder pain. The best course of action is to strive to have a healthy weight, and learn to strengthen your muscles using proper exercises in order to try and increase the endurance and strength in your back and help reduce pain. You might also consider therapeutic exercises to help alleviate pain. These tend to be less focused on building strength and more focused on alleviating pain and releasing tension. You can learn more about them in chapter 9.

Fashion

Fashion is an often unexpected culprit of back, neck, and shoulder pain. There are many types of fashion that can contribute to these pains, and a lot of them are popular in the modern world. High heel shoes, shoes without proper support, purses, bags, and other types of fashion can all contribute to a poor posture, resulting in back, neck, and shoulder pain. If you find that your pain is stemming from fashion choices, the best opportunity to alleviate pain is to eliminate these items from your wardrobe, and start practicing exercises that will help correct your posture and eliminate posture-related pains.

Stress

Stress itself can actually lend to back, neck, and shoulder pain. When we are stressed, we tend to subconsciously clench muscles in these areas. Chronic stress can result in us clenching these muscles for long periods of time, making it difficult for us to unclench them. As a result, we can be left with major knots and muscle pain. The best course of action for those dealing with back, neck or shoulder pain as a result of stress is to get to the root cause of the stress and eliminate it. Then, they should practice therapeutic exercises that will help their muscles release tension and help them relax once again.

There are many reasons why people tend to experience back pain. These are the most common ones, so you are likely to find your source of pain on this list. Remember, before you get into the exercises and actually alleviating this pain, you need to find the root cause of why it is happening. The best opportunity for you to truly relieve your back, neck, or shoulder pain is to diagnose it properly and then choose the relief methods that are unique to that type of pain. Otherwise, you may be treating the wrong symptoms, or simply covering the symptoms with pain medicines like many traditional doctors tend to do.

Chapter 3:
All About TMS in the Mind and Body

Tension Myositis Syndrome, or TMS, is a mind-body syndrome that causes pain in the body as a result of the brain function. This type of pain is not the result of injury, poor posture, or other physical influences. Instead, it is the brain causing the pain.

Manifesting of TMS

TMS manifests itself in many different forms. It may show up as back and leg pain, neck, shoulder and arm pain, or pain in the tendons. You may also have symptoms such as TMJ, and myofascial pain dysfunction, as well as fibromyalgia, myofacsical pain syndrome, carpal tunnel, and repetitive stress injuries. Post-polio syndrome, Epstein-Barr Virus, chronic fatigue syndrome, and many different types of chronic pain are also all manifestations of TMS.

Those who struggle with TMS may feel symptoms of pain, stiffness, tingling, muscle contractures, numbness, weakness, cramps, or any other painful sensations. The pain is primarily felt in the neck, back, wrists, knees and arms. The symptoms may move from body part to body part, making it difficult to identify exactly what hurts since it can change rapidly. This particular symptom: the moving of the pain, tends to be the primary indicator that someone may have TMS.

Psychology of TMS

TMS pain does not begin as a result of any physical cause or explanation. Instead, it is caused in the mind. This does not mean that the pain is all in your head, but rather that your mind is responsible for the real, physical pain that you are feeling in your body.

In TMS, it is believed that pain symptoms are actually caused by the autonomic nervous system mildly depriving the brain of oxygen. This happens when someone has a significant amount of repressed emotions, or psycho-social stress.

Ultimately, TMS is the result of excessive psychological stress on a person. This may be due to a desire to strive for perfectionism, trauma, anxiety, depression, and other difficult emotions. In society, we are often taught to repress anything that doesn't feel good. This, however, is the type of stuff that leads to TMS.

Physiology of TMS

The physiology of TMS is ultimately the fact that your brain mildly deprives oxygen to certain areas of the body when excessive amounts of stress are present. As a result, you can have a variety of different symptoms that stem from not having enough oxygen to certain areas of your body. These symptoms are exactly what we have talked about in the manifesting of TMS section of this chapter.

When you have TMS, there are no physically contributing factors to the pain you are experiencing. Physical traumas, postures, structural abnormalities and other conditions are not the cause of your back pain.

Instead, it is caused by psychological factors that are often overlooked by doctors. In modern medicine, psychiatrists focus on your mind and doctors focus on your body. There are very few people connecting the links between the two to consider how they uniquely work together and affect one another.

Treating TMS

The best way to treat TMS is to resume having a normal lifestyle, while also looking for ways to alleviate your emotional burdens and stress. Educating yourself on TMS and on emotional wellbeing, as well as working to truly resolve your emotional difficulties is important in order to alleviate the physical manifestations of what originally began as psychological pain.

If you are struggling to recover from your pain, you should consider attending psychotherapy or group treatment to help. The ultimate goal is to find the unique method that works best for you to help you truly heal your emotional struggles and traumas. As a result, you will see great improvement in your TMS symptoms.

It is important to understand that many people don't even realize they have TMS. Since they attend a doctor, who is primarily focused on finding physical conditions, they are driven in circles around what might be wrong. Often, they are handed a diagnosis that is not definitive or even truly proven. Instead, the doctor simply can't find what it is so they categorize it with something else the best they can. As a result, the patient (you) continues to feel many of the symptoms, regardless of the types of pain prescriptions provided. If this sounds like you, then you may want to consider treating yourself for TMS.

Chapter 4: Posture

As you learned in chapter 2, posture can be a major contributing factor when it comes to having back pain. Many people are unaware of what healthy posture is, and are unaware of the fact that it can change. Changing weights, age, and changing your orientation between standing, sitting, and lying down can all contribute to back pain as a result of poor posture.

How Posture Affects Your Back, Neck, and Shoulders

Our back, neck, and shoulders are built with muscles that are designed to help us with many things. Of these things include standing, sitting, and lying down. When we get lazy in our posture, we tend to put stress on these muscles in a way that is unnatural to how they are built. For example, when standing, the most common tendency is to slouch. This results in our back being curved in an unnatural manner which puts pressure on our lower back, shoulders, and neck. After prolonged periods in these unhealthy postures, we begin to feel pain in these areas as a result of this pressure.

Poor posture can result for many reasons. It may result due to laziness or a lack of education on what proper posture looks like. It can also result in additional weight on the body, either through body fat or external sources such as carrying heavy bags around on a regular basis. We may also get it as a result of wearing fashion items, such as high heels or shoes that lack support. Regardless of how it occurs, posture-oriented pain can all be felt in the same areas: the back, neck, and shoulders. You may also feel pain in your joints and muscles in other areas of the body, such as your feet and legs, depending on where your poor posture begins.

How to Get Good Posture

Good posture starts in the feet. When standing, your feet should be shoulder width apart. The weight of your body should be evenly spread across your feet, not being carried on the fronts, backs, or sides of your feet. Your knees should be directly above your feet, and your hips above your knees. Your tailbone should be straight above your hips, then your back straight with your shoulders pulled back so that they are evenly across from each other and stacked over your hips. Your head should be straight up, not tilted forward or backward. Ultimately, your body should be stacked properly so that each part is supporting the surrounding parts of your body.

Tricks to Eliminate Posture-Related Back Pain

The first step is to correct your posture, and eliminate any external influences that may be causing poor posture. For example, if you tend to wear high heels or improperly supported shoes, consider eliminating these from your wardrobe and purchasing supportive shoes that help you evenly spread your weight across your feet and feel comfortable doing so. You should also consider eliminating chairs that do not support your posture if you find yourself sitting in them for long periods of time, such as your office chair. Instead, replace them with an ergonomic chair that features support for your entire back and helps you stay in the appropriate position that keeps your posture strong.

You should also regularly switch between standing and sitting throughout the day. If you work in a job that requires you to sit for long periods of time, get up periodically for breaks. Walk around for a few minutes and stretch your body out, while maintaining proper standing posture. If you stand frequently at your job, take regular sitting breaks. Sit down and ensure that you maintain proper sitting posture, while giving your legs, hips, and back a break from the burden of standing for long periods of time.

You should regularly check your posture to see if you are maintaining a proper and supportive posture. Be sure to check your posture when you are sitting, standing, driving, walking, and during any other regular activity. You want to do your best to maintain a strong posture at all times, regardless of what activity you are engaging in. The more you are in a proper posture, the more you are going to train your body to maintain that posture and alleviate your pain associated with having a poor posture.

If your posture is a result of weight, you should consider where the added weight is coming from. If it is from weight gain, do your best to eliminate the weight you are carrying. If it is from carrying a bag around for many hours a day, look for one that distributes the weight more evenly across your body, and that features proper support to help you carry it more efficiently. You should also look to eliminate as much unnecessary weight from it as possible.

Sometimes people who have had poor posture for a long period of time have very tight and sore muscles when they begin to correct their posture. If this is the case, you may feel a lack of desire to correct your posture as a result of the pain you are feeling. To correct it properly, go slow and correct it a bit at a time. Also, do exercises that will help strengthen your muscles and release any residual tension you may be feeling in them. This will help ensure that you are not feeling constant pain in your back as a result of attempting to correct your posture, and will encourage you to continue working towards achieving a healthy posture.

Chapter 5:
Improper Treatment and Diagnosis

Recently, the way back pain was handled is incredibly dysfunctional. The pain is viewed as a condition in and of itself, and many different types of pain medicines are prescribed as a means to help alleviate the pain. As a result, many people are having a symptom of a larger problem treated as if it were the only problem, which leads to improper treatment methods, undiagnosed conditions, and worsening symptoms as a result.

The biggest problem with these diagnosis and treatment methods is not only that they don't work, but that many people are prescribed medicines that potentially create larger issues. The most common medicines to be prescribed are opioids, and these have been proven to worsen conditions if not used properly.

Opioids are meant to help with severe pain for a short amount of time. When properly used, they are prescribed for treatment immediately after surgery or a major injury, and then something more mild is used for ongoing treatment until the pain is alleviated. Unfortunately, many doctors have been prescribing these as long-term pain treatment medications for years.

The reason why opioids are not intended for long term use is because people become tolerant to them, and then they become dependent. This leads to addictions, which can lead to increased pain symptoms and withdrawal symptoms. What the medicine is intended to heal actually becomes worse when these medicines are used for a long period of time.

There are many other types of pain medications that are prescribed, each of which comes with their own unique set of symptoms and conditions to look out for. While most don't cause the type of addictions opioids cause, they do cause other unwanted symptoms. Of these symptoms include things such as: deterioration of stomach lining, burning in the esophagus, constipation or diarrhea, nausea, sleepiness, and other symptoms that can be damaging or difficult to live with.

Another unfortunate side effect of using pain medicine is that it does not actually cure the problem. This means that you may "feel" better, but actually be worsening the condition because you are under the illusion that everything is well. For example, if you have an injury in your back and you take pain medicine, you may believe that you can lift heavier items than you actually should be. As a result of being under the illusion that you are not in pain, you are actually worsening the condition instead of improving it.

There are many reasons why pain medicines should not be used as a long-term care option, but unfortunately most doctors rely on this as their primary solution when it comes to treating back pain. Because there can be such an extensive number of reasons why someone is experiencing chronic back pain, and in many instances the ailment is a part of the mind-body connection and not just the mind or the body, many doctors never actually find the cause of the pain their patients are experiencing.

While taking pain medicines is certainly necessary in some conditions, it should not be used as a long-term option unless absolutely necessary. It is common that many doctors prescribe pain medicines and use them as a long-term care solution for their patients because they cannot think of alternatives that will actually serve their patient and prevent them from experiencing recurring pain. The remaining chapters in this book are going to explore the importance of understanding the cause of your pain, and choosing proper treatment solutions that will actually cure you from your pain, instead of merely covering it up and causing further ailments in the long run. These alternative therapies are proven to work, and have shown to have incredibly positive impacts on those who use them. In chapter 6 you are going to learn how you can treat your back pain based on the unique reason why you are suffering, and why it is important to choose a unique course of action that is going to serve your individual needs.

Chapter 6: Treating Back Pain

As you know, the best opportunity to treat back pain is to first understand where the root of the problem lies. Once you do, you can begin to create an action plan to help you find solutions on how you can solve your back pain.

In chapter 3 we explored many of the common causes of back pain, but now we are going to explore how you can determine what the cause of your back pain truly is. This can sometimes be easy to identify: if you notice you have particularly poor posture, for example, you can likely sum it up to your posture. However, if you feel that your poor posture is a result of something deeper, or you are unsure of what the underlying cause is, there are some things you can consider in order to get your pain properly diagnosed.

The first step of action is to rule out things that are easy to diagnose without much medical intervention. TMS, poor posture, stress, and other similar things can typically be easily identified by paying attention to your daily lifestyle and noticing if these particular ailments appear to stand out or not. If they do, you can easily start treating yourself for these using a series of different exercises and practicing proper posture. If they do not, however, you may have to go a little further.

The next step is typically exploring magnetic resonance imaging, commonly known as an MRI. This is a scan that produces detailed pictures of your body, allowing doctors to explore whether there may be any underlying issues. In some cases, people with severe back pain get MRI's as an opportunity to identify any physical issues that may be taking place and causing the pain. It is through MRI's that doctors can often diagnose structural issues that may be leading to you experiencing severe pain in your back, neck, or shoulders.

If you do get an MRI, you will then have a clear answer as to what you need to do in order to correct your pain. If they find nothing physically wrong, then you can assume that your pain is coming from something such as poor posture or stress. If they do, however, then you can discuss other solutions with your doctor.

Structural abnormalities can lead to back pain, but they don't always mean that back pain will be present. If you have a structural abnormality that is not considered to be extensive or extremely damaging, you might consider trying therapeutic exercises and strengthening exercises to correct the pain on your own before exploring medical options. However, if your pain is too severe, the abnormality is extensive, or your exercising is not helping, you and your doctor may consider exploring surgery as an opportunity to correct the area that is causing pain.

Choosing whether or not to do surgery is entirely unique to each individual situation. It is generally considered to be a last attempt at solving the problems individuals face with back pain. If you find that you are really struggling, that your own natural efforts are not helping, and that you are tired of taking medicine, it may be time to consider getting a surgery done. Remember, surgery will take time to heal from, so you will continue to feel pain until you are healed from your surgery. During that time, you will likely have to complete physio therapy, as well as take pain medicines that will help you recover from the surgery itself. If you are planning on getting this surgery, be prepared to be in healing mode for some time before you can resume your normal lifestyle.

If you find out that you are in pain and it is not related to a structural abnormality, or your abnormality is not extensive enough to require surgery, then it is time to consider alternative treatments. While pain medicines can be helpful, the ultimate goal is for you to recover from your pain enough that you no longer require these medicines. Remember, there is a fine line between using them to help for pain, and using them because you are dependent on them. You do not want to become dependent on them, because this can lead to a whole other world of issues.

Some people consider using steroids as treatment for back pain, but this is not advised. While some doctors believe it can be helpful, and it may cause short bursts of relief in pain, but it may not even give that. Many people report getting steroid treatments and feeling very little amounts of relief. When it comes to spinal conditions, it is shown that steroid treatments don't actually help, and therefore they are simply a waste of time while adding foreign bodies to your system that may have negative side effects for those who get them.

Better forms of remedy include proper exercises, correcting your posture, and many varieties of traditional Chinese medicine that has been shown to improve back pain. There is an extensive list of alternative therapies you can attempt as an opportunity to heal your back pain and allow you to resume a pain free life. These remedies have proven they are capable of treating all types of back pain, from TMS and stress-induced pain, to pain associated with structural abnormalities, and all other types of pain.

When it comes to deciding what methods you should use to heal your back pain, you really have to consider where your pain is coming from and the severity of it. For example, if you have severe back pain as a result of muscle tension and stress, you might want to start with relaxing and therapeutic exercises, as well as gentle strength-building exercises that will assist you with increasing the strength in your muscles and releasing the tension and stress.

If you have pain as a result of an injury or physical trauma to your back, you may consider using something further such as massage, Qi, acupuncture, chiropractic care, yoga, and other similar treatments. You should also consider the fact that most back pain therapies and treatments actually require for individuals to combine two or more of the alternative methods to really experience full relief from their pain.

Treating back pain comes in three levels: diagnosing the cause, curing the cause, and maintaining a pain free life. It is important that once you have diagnosed the reason for your pain and found solutions that assist you in treating it, that you continue with these solutions. Back pain, especially the chronic kind, can settle back in when we are not careful. It is important that you understand that once you have alleviated the worst of your pain, you must maintain some form of plan in place to prevent your back pain from returning.

In most cases, prevention requires the sufferer to continue with light to moderate exercises on a regular basis. Strengthening the back, shoulder and neck muscles and using them regularly can have a significant impact on one's ability to prevent pain from returning. There are many exercises you can use as an opportunity to eliminate your pain, which you will learn about in Chapter 8. Additionally, you can use alternative therapies and medicines like acupuncture, medicine and chiropractic care as an opportunity to ward off any flare ups you may have if you find that your pain is returning despite maintaining a regular exercise regimen.

Treating back pain is something that requires diligent attention and care. This is why most people end up suffering for many years, or using pharmaceutical medicines and addictive pain medications to help them with the pain. Despite every day doctors doing their best to help with pain management, many are unaware of the alternative therapies that individuals can use as a solution to cure back pain. They figure that if they can "treat" the problem with a simple medication, then everything must be better. Unfortunately, as a sufferer, this can be a struggle. You may find yourself wanting to have better pain management systems, not wanting to use addictive medications that may not even entirely work, and wanting to have a long term solution that is better than merely taking daily medicines or pain pills as necessary.

Chapter 7: Traditional Healing Methods

Popular medicine presently relies heavily on prescription medications as a solution to heal back pain, when in reality these don't actually heal the pain at all. Instead, they simply lead individuals to *feel* healed and experience some relief, without actually healing the cause of the pain at all. Traditional healing methods are based on healing the common reasons why people suffer from back pain, which tend to cover all of the bases.

There are four extremely common traditional medical therapies you can use, as well as many other traditional methods you can use as an opportunity to heal your back pain and prevent yourself from feeling it ever again. In this chapter, we will cover all of those remedies.

Chiropractic Care

When used, chiropractic alignments have proven extremely successful in helping alleviate many different causes of back pain. Chiropractic care involves a trained practitioner readjusting your back using special massage-like techniques that put your bones back into place. When we stand with poor posture, lift things frequently, and even engage in regular daily activities, we tend to slowly move our backs out of alignment. As a result, we may experience severe pain in our backs. Getting a chiropractic alignment will help realign the parts of your back that are thrown out by regular daily activity, and help reduce the amount of pain you are feeling. Many report positive benefits from using this type of therapy to help their back.

When it comes to chiropractic care, the amount of time it will take for you to feel relieved from your pain will vary. Most users report feeling significant improvement immediately after one session, and the amount of improvement continues to increase after each session. Most users find that they require between 3 and 5 sessions to feel completely better, depending on the severity of their pain and how far out of alignment their back was. Chiropractic practitioners will not completely align a severely misaligned back all in one session, as this can lead to further pain from the sufferer. Instead, they will do it slowly over a series of sessions until you are returned to a fully aligned state. They then return for chiropractic care every 6-12 months as an opportunity to maintain the alignment and prevent themselves from experiencing severe pain again.

Acupuncture

Acupuncture is a widely talked about method to help alleviate back pain that can have a significantly impact on healing back, neck, and shoulder pain. The practice involves a practitioner inserting small, sterilized needles into specific points in your back, neck, and shoulders. Acupuncture has been practiced as a part of traditional Chinese medicine for more than 2,500 years. They claim there are over 2000 points on the body where these needles can be inserted for relief. The majority of people who seek acupuncture care are those suffering with chronic back pain, and most report that they experience significant improvement in their pain following their treatments.

Some wonder if acupuncture is safe or not, since you are being tapped with small needles in a variety of places around your back, neck, and shoulders. When you attend an experienced, licensed, and qualified practitioner, you can feel confident that you are not going to be at risk for experiencing any side effects. Infections, punctured organs, and other side effects are highly rare, and typically only occur as a result of visiting an unqualified practitioner who is not actually practiced in this type of treatment.

Acupuncture is one type of treatment that should be discussed with your doctor, as those who are pregnant, have a pacemaker, have an implant, or take certain types of medication should avoid this type of treatment. Additionally, your doctor may be able to refer you to an acupuncture practitioner to help you get set up with a reputable person who will do a good job.

Like with chiropractic care, most sufferers must visit several times before they are completely healed from their pain. However, you should experience significant improvement after every session. Users typically report needing 3-5 sessions before they experience complete relief from their pain, though they may go on an ongoing basis in order to maintain this relief.

Massage

For those who have back pain as a result of tension, stress, or overworked muscles, they may consider getting a massage to help relieve their symptoms and heal themselves from back pain. Massage tends to be a great solution for those who have chronic back pain as a result of both physical tension and overworked muscles, and mental stress and discomfort. It is known to have a therapeutic effect on both the body and mind.

There are a variety of massages that may be considered for chronic back pain, though the most commonly chosen variety is known as a deep tissue massage. Deep tissue massages are excellent at helping work out knots and tension that are built up in the back muscles and relieve an individual of this type of pain. They generally last around an hour, and most types of tension can typically be entirely worked out in this hour long session. Some will go back for two or three, however, if they are experiencing significant amounts of pain from stress and tension in their back.

Because of their therapeutic effect on both the mind and body, massages tend to be used as a regular ongoing form of treatment when individuals are wanting to relieve themselves from pain. They are great for helping relieve individuals from mental stress and discomfort, as well as physical pain and discomfort.

One important thing to note is that if you have a physical injury or trauma to your back, you must notify your masseuse of this condition. There are many conditions that can actually be worsened by massage therapy, so you want to be sure that you are not exposing yourself to greater pain and actually worsening the condition. It is imperative that you are open and honest with your practitioner to avoid being further injured.

Yoga

Yoga is an incredible form of exercise to help individuals who are experiencing back pain as a result of tension or stress. It can also be beneficial to those who have minor injuries in the back, though you want to be careful not to overdo it and worsen your injury. If you have extensive injuries, there may be some extremely easy exercises you can do to help you start getting strength back, but it will heavily depend on the severity of your injury and the symptoms you are facing as a result.

Yoga is a low-impact type of workout that enables individuals to strengthen muscles while also stretching them out and getting some relief from tension. It can serve in many ways, and can also be directed towards different goals. For example, there are certain yoga moves you may favor if you are looking to build strength, and others you might favor if you are looking to release tension and extend your range of movement and flexibility.

The idea behind yoga is to use it as a regular part of your maintenance routine. It will certainly help alleviate initial pain, but is also excellent for helping keep pain at bay. Yoga is wonderful for many reasons, including increasing strength and flexibility, alleviating symptoms of pain especially when related to tension or stress, increasing circulation, and helping individuals have an overall greater sense of wellbeing. People who use yoga as a means to alleviate existing pain typically use it on a regular basis and see improvement in their symptoms in as little as one week. By one month, most of their symptoms tend to be gone.

Diet

Many people are unaware that there are actually many different parts of your diet that can influence pain. Certain diets can lead to inflammatory issues, which can mean that various areas in your back are inflamed, also. If you are experiencing pain in many areas around your muscles and joints, you may be struggling with mild to moderate inflammation. Altering your diet can greatly improve your ability to eliminate pain associated with inflammation. Furthermore, there are certain things you can eat that help with pain in general. These foods contain various nutrients that act like supplements and can help your body ward off pain. People who use diet as a means to manage pain typically use it in conjunction with other pain-management methods, so it is hard to say how much or how quickly you will experience relief from pain using this method alone, but it has been proven to be an effective add-on to an existing pain management system.

When managing pain through diet, you want to avoid consuming anything that may have sugar, alcohol, caffeine, or trans fats in them. These are all known for increasing inflammation and pain in individuals, which can go against the purpose of your pain management system. Eating high fiber foods, foods that are rich in potassium, omega-3 fats, and clean lean proteins are helpful. You should also increase your water intake, as it can help flush your body of harmful and unwanted toxins.

Supplements

In addition to changing your diet, there are many supplements that have been reported to have an incredibly positive impact when it comes to relieving pain symptoms. These supplements each work for unique reasons, so we will explore them further below. People who add these supplements report greater benefits from their pain-management system and relief in as little as two weeks. With some supplements you will want to consult your doctor, as they may not pair well with any medications you may presently be on, or any health concerns or conditions you may have.

Fish Oil (2,000mg Daily) is known to reduce inflammation. For the same reason it is helpful in your diet, it is also helpful when you take it as a supplement. Taking it in supplement form helps you increase the amount you are consuming to a level higher than you can likely comfortably consume from your regular diet.

Turmeric (1,000mg Daily) has been reported to have wonderful healing benefits when it comes to pain and inflammation. The active ingredient in this supplement is curcumin, which has powerful anti-inflammatory agents in it, helping heal and reduce pain you may be experiencing.

Proteolytic Enzymes (Bromelain and Papain) (500mg, 3x per Day) is naturally found in pineapple, and has a very strong ability to help reduce inflammation and pain. Many people also state that you can regularly consume pineapple juice in order to gain the same benefits.

MSM (2,000-8,000mg Daily) has been known to help reduce pain, since it is a strong anti-inflammatory supplement. This supplement is high in sulfur, which helps rebuild cartilage and eliminate symptoms such as muscle spasms.

Magnesium (400-500mg Daily) is used for helping with pain associated with muscles. Many individuals claim you can also drink coconut milk or coconut water for the same effect, since both are also rich in magnesium. This supplement helps relax muscles and can reduce tension and stress that builds up in them. It may cause diarrhea, however, so decrease your dosage if you experience this symptom.

Walking

Walking and other types of light cardio are a great way to help alleviate back symptoms that are associated with posture, stress, tension, and otherwise tense muscles. When you walk on a regular basis, particularly when you swing your arms in large and defined swings, you help move the muscles in your back. In modern life, we don't often move these muscles in the ways that we should, so they can become tense and stiff. If you walk more regularly, especially with a healthy walking posture, you can help release the tension you feel in this area and therefore decrease the amount of pain as well.

Alternatives to walking include cycling and aerobic swimming. These types of low-impact cardio are great for working out your body and muscles while increasing your circulation and helping heal muscles in your back that may be tense or stressed out. Be careful using these if you are experiencing pain as a result of an injury, because you do not want to worsen it.

People who use walking or other forms of light cardio to alleviate back pain report feeling relief from symptoms in as little as one week. In addition to feeling relief from back pain, they also report a greater sense of wellbeing overall. These types of activity are known to improve mental endurance, mood, and physical stamina and wellbeing. They have a very positive impact overall and should be considered as a part of your pain-management system.

Essential Oils

Essential oils are often a controversial topic, as many people report that they are not beneficial and others claim they are incredible. There is actually a great deal of science behind the chemistry in essential oils and how they work, so they can be considered proven as a relief system for many who are experiencing back pain.

When it comes to essential oils, you want to pick ones that are known to be analgesics, as this means that they work directly on pain. Peppermint and wintergreen oils are both incredible choices for this purpose. You should dilute one to two drops of these oils into a carrier oil like fractionated coconut oil or jojoba oil and massage them into the areas that hurt most. Be sure not to use more than 5 drops if you are a healthy adult, as they can be strong and have negative side effects if you use too much. You should consult your doctor as well as a certified aromatherapist if you are elder, under the age of 18, or have a medical condition, as they will be able to help ensure you get the proper dose that will not impose a threat to your health or safety.

There are many methods that you can use to heal back pain. Instead of using conventional medicines that are often full of harsh chemicals that can be damaging if used long-term, these methods are more holistic and provide a greater sense of relief. Furthermore, they can help get to the root cause of your ailment and provide true relief by actually healing the ailment you are suffering with, instead of merely hiding it beneath pain pills, steroids, and opioids. In addition to these methods, you should also add a regular exercise routine to your daily pain-management system. In chapter 8 we will explore various exercises you can use to help eliminate back pain, depending on how severe it is and your abilities.

Chapter 8:
Exercises to Alleviate Symptoms

Exercise is known to be one of the best ways to alleviate pain symptoms in the back, neck, and shoulders. Most pain in these areas exists as a result of muscle tension and muscle stiffness, so exercising can help release the tension and strengthen these muscles to avoid further pain.

While you are reading this section, be sure to mind the true reason why you are in pain. If you have suffered an injury or have a physical condition causing the pain, be sure to go over your exercise plan with a doctor who can confirm that your plan will not cause further harm to you in your condition. You want to be sure that you are paying attention to your physical wellbeing and that you are promoting it, rather than further damaging yourself. Be sure that if anything ever hurts, feels uncomfortable, or causes any type of further pain, that you stop immediately. While many of these exercises are intended to build strength, they are not intended to cause prolonged pain. You should not feel excessive pain in the moment, nor in the days following your exercise. If you do, stop immediately and consult your doctor or health care practitioner.

These exercises are broken down by area targeted, but you should use a selection of exercises from each section that you are struggling with to create your own unique exercise plan that will help you alleviate pain all over your back, neck, and shoulders. This will ensure that all areas in question are targeted and you are alleviated from the pain you have been struggling with.

Exercises for Neck Pain

Your neck is a very sensitive area, so you always want to be sure that you are being extra gentle with it. While any sore muscle should be treated with care, your neck muscles tend to be extra delicate so you want to be extremely cautious when exercising your neck to alleviate pain.

There are six really good stretches you can try that are known to help decrease the pain you feel in your neck. These are great for when you are actively feeling pain, and to prevent pain.

Seated Neck Release

This is an extremely easy exercise where you sit on the ground with your legs crossed and put your left hand on the floor next to you. Then, with your right hand, reach over and grab the left side of your head and gently pull it to the right. Don't pull until it hurts, just pull until you feel a stretching sensation. Hold this for a few minutes and then release. Repeat on the other side.

Seated Clasping-Hand Neck Stretch

From the same position as your seated neck release, you can clasp your hands together and place them at the base of your skull. Gently pull your head forward until your chin comes close to your chest. Don't feel as though you have to touch chin to chest, but do pull it in this direction. This will help you release tension in the back of your neck.

Behind the Back Neck Stretch

Standing with your feet shoulder width apart, evenly spread your weight across your feet. Then, reach behind your back and grab your left wrist with your right hand. Pull your shoulders back and then press your right ear towards your right shoulder. After about 5-10 seconds, gently roll your head to the other side and push your left ear towards your left shoulder. Release.

Grounded Behind the Back Tuck Stretch

For this stretch, you want to get on the ground on your hands and knees. Evenly distribute your weight across your knees, and have them placed firmly under your hips so that you aren't shifting during the stretch. Then, place the top of your head on the ground, and gently put your hands behind your back, clasping them together. Straighten your arms and send them straight up behind your back so that your back, shoulders, and neck are all getting a really good stretch. Do not use this stretch if you are experiencing severe pain because it could lead to stress on the muscles and further pain. This is for those with mild pain or tension, or who are looking to maintain a pain-free lifestyle following the elimination of existing pain entirely.

Seated Open Heart Stretch

For this stretch, you want to sit on your knees with your bum on your heels and your toes pointing straight back. Then, you want to reach your arms back about one foot behind your feet and place your hands firm on the floor with your fingers pointing away from your body. Lean back so that your shoulders are over your hands, and press your chest up into the sky. Hold this for about 15-20 seconds before releasing. Repeat about 3 more times.

Bridge

The bridge is a great pose for releasing neck pain. To get into it, you want to sit on the ground with your knees up in front of you. Then, lay back so that your shoulders are on the floor. Tuck them in so that they are tucked under your back. Then, reach your hands down behind your back and clasp them together under your bum. When you are ready, push your hips up into the air. Your body should be a straight diagonal line from your shoulders up to your knees. Hold this pose for about 20 seconds before releasing. Repeat about 3 more times.

Exercises for Shoulder Pain

Shoulder pain can be a result of neck and upper back pain, or it can be the cause of it. Either way, you want to make sure that you are exercising properly to help eliminate the pain in these areas. There are many excellent shoulder exercises you can do to eliminate tension and pain in these areas, including the following six. Some of these exercises require some type of light weight or an elastic exercise band, but you may improvise without these if you are dealing with excessive pain or an injury.

Shoulder Rotations

Stand with your feet shoulder width apart and evenly distribute your weight across them. Then, pull your shoulders up towards your ears and start rotating them in clockwise circles, keeping your arms by your side. After about 15 rotations, switch to a counter-clockwise position and do it for another 15 rotations. Next, place your arms directly out beside you and start rotating your arms in a tight, clockwise rotation for about 15 rotations. Then, reverse and go in the opposite direction. Continue doing this, gradually increasing your circles as you go, until you are doing it with large drawn out circles.

Shoulder Doorway Stretch

Stand in front of a doorway and place your arms directly out on either side of you. Move forward so that your arms are touching the door frame, and ensure you are evenly in the middle so the same part of each arm is touching the door frame. Then, walk forward through the door slowly and gently, so that your arms are pressed behind you. Hold for about 15 seconds before releasing. Repeat about 3 more times, or as needed to release pain in the shoulders.

Side-Lying Rotation

Lay on the floor on your side, with your head propped up by your elbow and your knees out at a 90-degree angle in front of you. With the hand on the top of your body (the right hand if you are laying on your left side, the left hand if you are laying on your right side,) grab a light weight and start rotating your arm at a 90-degree angle, from the floor to straight up in the air above you. Your elbow should be bent at a 90-degree angle so that the weight is being lifted up over the top of you from directly in front of you. Repeat about 10-15 sides on one side before turning over to do the same on the other side.

High-to-Low

Put one knee on the ground and one foot out in front of you, like a resting lunge pose. Your knee should be directly under your hip, and your shoulders should be directly over your hip. Then, reach the arm that is on the same side of your knee on the ground up in front of you at a diagonal angle from your body, make a fist and pull it back down. For added effect, you can attach an exercise band to something above you so that you are pulling the band every time you pull your arm back towards your body. Reposition yourself to complete the exercise on the opposite side. Do about 15 stretches per each side.

Reverse Fly

Stand with your knees shoulder length apart and evenly distribute your weight on each foot. Then, bend your knees slightly and lean forward so that your back is at a diagonal angle to the ground, with your head being at the highest point. Then, using a weight that is comfortable for you, hold one in each hand. Hold your hands together in front of your knees, then simultaneously move each one up so that your arms are straightened, without ever locking your elbows to have your arms fully straight. They should stay lightly bent to prevent injury. Push your hands back until they are slightly higher than your back, then bring them back together in front of your knees. Repeat 15-20 times.

Exercises for Upper Back Pain

When you have upper back pain, you typically want to combine exercises that target upper back pain with neck and shoulder exercises to get full relief. The following exercises will help you achieve that relief, in addition to a combination of exercises from the previous two sections.

Wall Stretch

Stand about two feet away from a wall, facing the wall. Reach your arms out and place your palms flat against the wall so that they are directly in front of your shoulders. Slowly walk your hands all the way down the wall until they are in front of your waist. Ensure your back stays straight. If necessary, step forward or back from the wall to create a 90-degree angle. Once you have created a 90-degree angle, roll your shoulders back and allow yourself to sway slightly so that you feel a stretch taking place in your upper back. Make sure your head stays upright, as you do not want it to hang down. This can create further pain, so it is important that your head stays upright. Hold your stretch for between thirty seconds and one minute before walking your hands up the wall and returning to your normal standing position.

Seated Stretch

Sit in a chair with your feet placed flat on the floor and your back straight up. Roll your shoulders back and press your shoulder blades down. Place your right palm on top of your right shoulder and your left palm on top of your left shoulder, with your elbows directly out to the sides. Once you are comfortable, move your elbows in front of you, trying to touch them together. Once you feel a good stretch in your upper back, stop and hold this position for 5 deep breaths. Release your elbows back to the side, then repeat the stretch about 10 times.

Yoga Strap Stretch

Sit on a chair with your feet planted on the floor in front of you. Hold a yoga strap or resistance band in front of you, with your arms locked straight and your palms facing forward. When you are ready, raise your hands directly above your head, keeping your elbows straight. Adjust your hands along the strap as necessary to be able to comfortably complete the stretch. With your arms above your head, lower your chin to your chest. Keep the strap taut and hold the position for about five deep breaths. Lower your arms back in front of you and repeat about 10 times.

Exercises for Lower Back Pain

Lower back pain can be extremely uncomfortable and can worsen as we walk or move. It can completely change the way we lead our lives, so you want to be sure that you are staying on top of lower back pain and working to heal it as much as possible. These exercises are great for relieving lower back pain, but you should be careful when exercising this part as it can easily become more agitated if you are not gentle and cautious.

Reverse Childs Pose

Reverse child's pose is an excellent, gentle way to release tension in your lower back. Start by laying on your back on the floor. Then, pull your knees up to your chest. Wrap your arms around your legs so that your hands come together in front of your knees, and pull your knees as close to your chest as you comfortably can. You should start to feel a stretch in your lower back. If you want, you can gently rock side to side in this pose to help further relieve tension in the lower back. Hold for about 30 seconds to 1 minute before releasing.

Partial Crunches

Lay on your back with your knees up in the air, about shoulder width apart. Put your hands across your chest to touch the opposite shoulders, or place your finger tips on your forehead. Very gently lift your shoulders up off the ground about 2-3 inches before releasing. Repeat about 10 times, or as many as you can comfortably handle. Do not do full sit ups if you experience lower back pain, as you can worsen your pain which is the opposite of what you want to accomplish!

Hamstring Stretches

Lay on your back with your knees up, as if you were about to do a partial crunch. When you are ready, straighten one leg out below you, and then lift it up into the air. If you need to, place a yoga band behind your calf to help you pull your leg straight up. Only pull until it feels comfortable, do not pull too far or you can worsen the pain and cause injuries to your muscles and ligaments. After about 5 deep breaths, release and repeat on the other side. Rotate back and forth for about 5 times on each side.

Cobra Pose

Lay on your stomach with your legs out behind you and your toes on the ground. Bend your arms so your elbows are tucked in next to your hips and your hands are at your shoulders. When you are ready, press your chest up in the air, putting your weight onto your forearms. Keep your hips firmly on the ground, but push yourself up in the air as high as you comfortably can. Hold this pose for about 30 seconds to 1 minute before releasing.

Bird Dog

Get on the ground on your hands and knees. Ensure your hands are directly under your shoulders and your knees are directly under your hips. Your weight should be evenly distributed across all four. When you are ready, shift your weight so that you can lift one leg and extend it directly behind you. Hold it for about 5 seconds before releasing and repeating on the other leg. For added effect, you can hold your arms out, too. To accomplish this more advanced position of bird dog, you would want to extend your right leg and left arm at the same time, and your left leg and right arm at the same time. Alternate between the two sides about 5 times each.

Chapter 9: In Case of Emergency

If you are experiencing severe pain in your back, it is important that you take appropriate action. Emergencies to do with the back require medical care to ensure that you are treated appropriately for your condition and nothing worsens.

You can identify an emergency related to your back if you experience brand new pain that persists longer than three days, is unbearable, or occurs as a result of an injury you have endured to your back. It is important that you call the appropriate help line in the event of an emergency. If you are not concerned about your immediate health or safety, call your doctor and book an appointment for as soon as possible. Record your symptoms and experiences to ensure that you are being treated for everything that is wrong and that your doctor can treat you correctly. If you are concerned for your immediate health or safety, you should attend the emergency room at your local hospital to seek treatment.

Even though there are alternative healing methods that can and should be considered when it comes to back pain, it is important that you take it seriously and seek treatment when necessary. Alternative medicine is powerful and can help greatly in many ways, but when you are experiencing an emergency, proper medical care may be required. Having the care of your doctor or an emergency doctor can ensure that you are being diagnosed properly. Following your diagnosis, you can create an action plan to help you heal from your pain.

You should consider a situation an emergency if you are experiencing one of the following:

- Back pain accompanied by severe stomach pain
- Incapable of moving a leg at all
- Heart attack symptoms (such as chest pain or pressure, nausea, sweating, vomiting, shortness of breath, sudden weakness, light-headedness, irregular

heartbeat, and/or pain, pressure, or discomfort in jaw, back, neck, upper belly, or one or both arms.)

You should consider the situation one that should be attended to by a medical physician if you experience any of the following:

- New or worsening symptoms of pain in your limbs, back, shoulders, or neck
- Back pain accompanied by other unusual symptoms such as diarrhea, or loss of bladder or bowel control
- Back pain that resulted from an injury, or back pain following an injury that was previously treated
- Back pain that lasts longer than 4 weeks
- Back pain that is accompanied by unexplained weight loss
- Back pain that occurs after age 50
- You currently have or have previously had cancer

Being able to properly handle emergencies or medical situations is important. It is vital that you understand that alternative medicine is a powerful healing agent when it comes to helping heal a less-severe diagnosis, or when it is added as a part of a larger action-plan to heal and eliminate back pain. You should never ignore signs of an emergency or medical distress in favor of alternative care, as this can lead to undiagnosed conditions that may result in a much worse situation going forward.

PART II

Chapter 1: How to Choose the Right Number of Repetitions

"How do I choose the number of repetitions and series?"

This is one of the main doubts that assail the neophytes of the gym. I still remember the day I asked my gym instructor about it many years ago. In fact, the first questions that a beginner poses to the instructor in front of a weight machine are typically these: "How many consecutive lifts (or movements) do I have to do with this machines? And for how many times?"

The most precise ones even dare to ask how much time they have to recover from one set to the next one, and so you think you have clarified everything you need to know about a training session at a given weight machine.

The load (i.e., the kg lifted or moved) is generally fixed according to the presumed abilities of the aspiring visitor of the weight room, often without any relation to the first two parameters of repetitions and sets.

There is not a unique answer to these questions since it all depends on the goal. For example, when I first started my training journey, I wanted to get bigger, not stronger. During that period I did a lot of hypertrophy-oriented workouts which worked quite well. When I switched to a more strength-oriented approach, I had to completely rearrange my schedule all over again.

Since the weight training that interests us is not aimed at the practice of bodybuilding—but is framed in the health of those who want to integrate aerobic activities with exercises for the general improvement of strength, elasticity, and flexibility—before defining the number of repetitions and sets, it is necessary to establish the objective to be achieved or what aspect do you want to train for between the following:

- **The resistant force**: the force that the muscle must apply to overcome the fatigue resulting from a prolonged effort.

- **The maximal force**: the maximum force that the muscle can develop with a lifting test (or a limited number of tests). It is also often referred to as a maximal load if referring to a specific exercise in the gym.

- **The fast force:** the maximum force that the muscle can develop to counteract a load in a limited period of time. Referring to time, therefore, more than force we should speak of power which is the ability to develop a force in the unity of time.

- **Muscle hypertrophy**: no reference is made to the type of force that the muscle has to generate, but to its effect on the athlete's body—that is, to maximize the increase in muscle volume. The muscular volume is connected to the developed force, because the greater the cross section of the muscle, the greater the muscle fibers available to make the effort. However, the equation *muscle* *hypertrophy = greater muscle strength* is not always true because, in addition to having available muscle fibers, the human body must also know how to recruit, and this is influenced by other factors such as the efficiency of the cardio-respiratory system, the ability coordination, etc. This should make those who seek to maximize muscle hypertrophy think only of achieving the highest possible performance.

In a healthy view of strength training, you can leave out the last point because the search for muscle hypertrophy, typical of bodybuilders, is far from our goals. Therefore, we can identify three types of training, each of which corresponds to a type of strength that you want to train and, consequently, to a pattern of repetitions-number of sets-interval between the different series.

Remember that to define a training plan, the following variables must be defined for each exercise (i.e., for each machine in the gym or exercise with weights):

- Repetition: it is the single gesture of weightlifting or athletic gesture that stresses the muscle or a district of the muscles. Generally, in the gym at each repetition, the muscle or muscles lift or move a weight (load).

- Sets: the consecutive number of repetitions. The set can be slow or fast, or the exercise is done slowly, calmly, or quickly, imposing to adhere to a higher rhythm.

- Recovery: the time between one series and the next.

So, you might find a typical 3-row workout of 12 sets of 25 kg with a three-minute recovery. This is a very standard way to get started and the first style of training that I followed when started out.

Chapter 2: How to Breathe During Exercises

One thing that is often overlooked by many gym enthusiasts is how to perform proper breathing during weight exercises. It is a problem that, sooner or later, most of those who attend gyms propose to their instructor.

Breathing, as we know, is an activity that we do involuntarily, but it is also possible to control it trying to adapt the movement of the muscles (or part of the muscles) involved, such as the diaphragm, the ribcage, the shoulders, abdominals to the rhythm that we want to follow.

Consciously, one can control the inhalation phase and the exhalation phase in their overall duration or even suspend breathing by entering apnoea.

A lot of sports and disciplines (yoga, pilates, etc.), give a lot of importance to breathing, while other oriental disciplines even give it a spiritual value.

Even in the exercises that are performed in the gym, including those with weights, breathing has a considerable importance. Unfortunately, there are not many who have clear ideas about it.

Instructors usually advise to:

- **inhale** in the discharge phase of the action, usually when the weight is being returned to its initial position;

- **exhale** in the loading phase of the exercise or when there is more effort required.

This usually works well, even if the beginner will at first see this as another constraint which will only confuse him. In reality, it requires a good amount of concentration to force yourself to control breathing in this way and therefore forces the athlete to give complete attention to what he is doing. A lot of times, people look around in the gym while doing an exercise, or—worse—talking to someone. This is something that I have never understood: to me, strength training is a way to become the best version of myself, both physically and mentally, and I do not have time to waste. Focusing on breathing is a good way to think exclusively about the exercise you are performing.

The following is a good general rule to follow:

The most important thing to do is not to hold your breath during the loading phase.

Holding your breath in the loading phase is a big mistake, as it is instinctive to hold your breath during the maximum effort required. Instead, the opposite must be done because this practice can also lead to serious consequences, especially if the effort involves muscles of the upper body.

Holding the breath deliberately blocks the glottis, which then leads to a compression of the veins due to an increase in pressure inside the ribcage. As a result of this compression, the veins can also partially occlude (as if they were strangled by one hand) and this considerably slows the return of venous blood to the heart. As a consequence, the arterial pressure rises, reaching even impressive values such as 300 mmHg (usually 120 mmHg at rest). Moreover, as a consequence of the reduced blood supply to the heart, the outgoing blood also slows down and reduces, which decreases the blood and oxygen supply to the peripheral organs. Less blood and oxygen to the brain could result in dizziness, blurred vision, etc. until you eventually faint. These are side effects well-known by opera singers who practice hyperventilation exercises that, in some parts, are performed in apnoea.

Chapter 3: Machines or Free Weights?

The question is interesting, and the purpose of this chapter is to precisely evaluate the advantages and disadvantages of two possible training solutions for muscle strengthening: the use of gym machines or exercise with the aid of free weights.

From a health point of view, it is clear that the question of the title seems reasonable because, unlike in a bodybuilder, muscle strengthening is seen only as a preparatory to a sport or as a general improvement of the body, and therefore it is not said that the use of gym machines is actually the only possible solution for those who want to make a good upgrade without wanting to reach professional levels of a bodybuilding lover. Before analyzing the two solutions in detail, briefly remember that a muscle can perform an effort in two ways of contraction: eccentric or concentric.

In the first case, the muscle develops the force necessary for the exercise when it is stretching, in the second case when it is being shortened.

Weights and machines are not always equivalent in stimulating a muscle in an eccentric and concentric way. For the purpose of training, eccentric work is the most difficult—to the point that it can also induce pain and muscle damage. It is therefore important that, by deciding which exercises to perform (with the machines or with the weights), it is clear (otherwise you can ask the instructor like I did at the beginning of my journey in the gym) which exercises stimulate the muscles more eccentrically, to introduce them gradually into the plan of training avoiding injuries.

Weight Machines

In the gym, there are usually many weight machines. Generally, except for the multi-function stations, each of them trains a specific muscular district or even a single type of muscle. The effort put in place by the muscles during the execution of the exercise must counteract two physical forces: the weight force and the force due to the friction of the weight that it moves (often along ropes or pulleys).

As a general rule of the mechanics involved in the use of weights, during the eccentric contraction, the friction force is subtracted from that of the weight, while during the concentric contraction this force is added.

Free Weights

They are called free-weight exercises because usually the weights are not tied to ropes or pulleys of the machines, but simply gripped or tied to the body (for example with anklets) and carried out only with the aid of weights such as dumbbells and barbells, which are often seen on sale in supermarkets. Surely, compared to a workout with machines, the one with free weights is easier to put in place. Often, it is not even necessary to attend a gym; a small home space equipped with a mat, a bench (if required by the exercises), a mirror (optional, to control the movements) and, of course, the weights is sufficient enough.

Now let's analyze the advantages and disadvantages of the two solutions, taking into consideration some objective parameters that can assume different importance depending on the individual's objectives, the physical state of departure (sedentary, beginner or advanced athlete), and the expectations placed in a training of this type.

- Economic aspect: free weight training is certainly cheaper, because, as mentioned, in most cases it is not necessary to get a gym subscription. It can be a good compromise solution to go to the gym for the time necessary to practice the exercises under the guidance of an experienced instructor, and then, once you are sure to perform the correct movements, buy weights and equip yourself with a training-space inside your home. This is what I did, and I would never go back.

- Versatility: free weights are suitable for multiple exercises and different muscle groups. Think about how many exercises you can do with simple weights to train biceps, triceps, pectorals, etc. In the case of training with weight machines, each machine usually allows a few exercises (if not only one) and this is the practical limit of such a training: you need to choose a gym where there is a sufficient number of machines for the exercises you want to do and where waiting times are not too long. Otherwise, the queues to the machines make the overall workout boring and ineffective.

- Eccentric and concentric training: weight machines usually lesser stress the eccentric work of the muscle (because of the opposing frictional force) unlike the movement of the body which, in returning to the starting position of the exercise, often performs eccentric work of considerable intensity. Moreover, in the exercises with weights, many antagonistic muscles are trained many times, and in general, they also train the balance and proprioceptive, improving body coordination.

- Safety and complexity: from the previous point, we can see that weight machines train specific muscle areas, and it is easier to isolate the muscle or muscle district involved. It is also easier to perform the exercise correctly because the movements are constrained by the machines and are easier to learn. With free weights, it is easier to make mistakes, and generally more antagonistic muscles and the spine are stimulated. In addition, with the weights, it is easier to maintain a constant execution speed. For all these reasons, it is generally said that the exercises with the machines are at a lower risk of injury than those with free weights.

Chapter 4: Putting it all together. How to program a training cycle

Now we come to the crucial point: how do I craft a strength training program? The question is very complex. Each strategy will be based on the condition of the subject, so, logically, when we see a disproportionate lack of strength for a muscle group, it will be logical to intervene in this sense. Let's go step by step. The literature on the subject highlights how, for the purposes of muscular hypertrophy and gains in strength, setting a periodized program is the best solution. Before diving deeper into the topic, it is important to note something. You cannot generalize, there is no way to use a unique approach or way of training a particular component. There are countless cases, solutions. So what can be done is to report different models based on different contexts to give not a guide but a concept—something infinitely more precious (and expendable).

Strategy 1. "Basic" Approach. A first approach that we can use is to set up a multifrequency workout by adopting a daily wavy periodization. So we will have two weekly sessions for each muscle district. In the first session we can train the muscle according to a traditional bodybuilding scheme, then longer TUT, intensity techniques, a range of 8-12 repetitions, eccentric, forced, etc. In the second session, we can train ourselves by adopting a progression of strength. So for example, we will train the chest on a flat bench using possibly another complementary exercise (like crosses, chest fly, etc.). A similar approach is at the base of the PHAT (Power Hypertrophy Adaptive Training) method proposed by

Norton. Unlike this, however, I find it more sensible to use—in training dedicated to strength—real progressions on exercises without being limited to a 5 × 5 standard type of training.

Strategy 2. Deficient Muscles Approach. Similar to the previous one, the only difference is that a workout in this sense will be done on the deficient muscles while the more developed muscles will be trained in mono-frequency. The increase in weekly volume and stimulus variation will bring an advantage in terms of growth (strength and hypertrophy) that will allow you to "catch up" with respect to the rest of the muscles. This approach can be used on deficient muscles both from a hypertrophy point of view and from a force point of view (i.e., the weakest muscles). This last aspect is particularly important as it can be a valid strategy to intervene where a muscle is placed limiting within the synergy of a gesture. The discourse can also be done from the opposite point of view—that is, to hold the strongest or most developed muscle groups to a multifrequency and to mono-frequency to recover asymmetries (aesthetic or functional).

Strategy 3. The transient phase of reduced volume. Another way to insert a strength training within a bodybuilding program is to provide a period with a high load intensity and a reduced volume. In this case, we always speak of wavy periodization. However, the variations will not be done on a daily basis, but weekly. So, for instance, we will put 2-3 up to 6 weeks of strength training with a reduced volume—less dense workouts but with the intensity of high-load and then return, progressively or not, to traditional bodybuilding sessions, or even to a wavy periodization protocol on a daily basis as described above. Basically, it is a matter of setting a transitional phase aimed at two purposes: Varying the stimulus (Ri) and finding the feeling with the motor scheme.

Strategy 4. Periodization within the session. This is also an interesting approach. It is a matter of inserting, within the session, an exercise on which to set up a forced schedule. In this sense, we could then insert the flat bench into a chest session as a first or second exercise. We will choose a program to improve on strength (since we are already able to exercise the right mastery over the exercise) and set the rest of the session as a traditional bodybuilding session. Obviously, the total volume will decrease as part of the session is occupied by dense work—not very voluminous but very intense. I find that such a setting fits well with the daily wavy periodization (strategy 1). Basically, by training a multi-frequency muscle, we will set the strength session using an exercise with its progression and the rest of the session in the traditional bodybuilding style. The diversification of work with respect to the second weekly session will be in the TUT (for example) which, in the latter, will be exasperated (e.g., +50'), while in the session of "strength" it will not be too high (e.g., 30').

Split and choice of exercises

A further aspect on which we must dwell is that relative to the decision, within the session, the target muscle groups and the exercises to be used. One of the characteristics of strength programs is that, in most cases, the various muscle groups are subdivided to work only a few each session. This is logical because the work that is required is always of the same type (anaerobic). Okay, as we have seen, it can work on different adaptive components, but in any case, it is always part of the big family of "boosting" work, the same that, in other sports, is alternated with "technical" work. The question that arises is the following: Should we first set the split and then, based on this, choose the type of exercises in which to work the strength or vice versa? Being a powerlifter myself, I would answer "the second," but from a Bodybuilder perspective I would answer "the first." Since this chapter is about strength training, I would say start from this context and, in particular, from the cases mentioned above. Where we want to set a wavy periodization, for all groups or only for some (strategies 1-2-4), then yes, we will have to start from the split. Based on this we will choose the best exercise on which to progress for the strength. So for example, in a push-day, we will choose the Bench Press for the chest, for a pull-day a Bent Over Row, and for a leg-day a Squat.

Let's do an example: Subject 1, Powerlifter, good management of high loads on the various motor schemes. Deficient groups: Arms, Back. Strong groups: Chest, Quadriceps

Split

Day 1 Push Day

Day 2 Pull Day

Day 3 Leg Day

Day 4 Rest

Day 5   Arms

Day 6   Back

Day 7   Glutes

Logically, we will then insert a progression on the Bent-Over Row on day 2 and work the Back with a traditional strength session on day 6. To evaluate a progression on the ground clearance that would be close to a leg workout (even putting it on day 6), we will have the hamstrings on day 7. But training strength, as we have seen, is not just a matter of periodizing and varying the stimulus, but also a question of functionality to the motor schemes to be performed during the sessions.

So let's take another example. Subject 2: Powerlifter, poor activation of the chest on the bench press, poor feeling on the deadlift. Excellent management of the Squat. Deficient groups: Chest-Back-Arms. The goal, in this case, will be to improve the feeling with easier exercises so we will set the split based on the same.

Split

Day 1   Chest and Shoulders

Day 2   Deadlift day

Day 3   Rest

Day 4   Quadriceps and Arms

Day 5   Rest

Day 6 Chest and Back

Day 7 Arms

Finally, in case we go set up a Strength program as a transitory phase (strategy 3), it will be logical to start from the exercises and, based on these, reason on the split.

PART III

Chapter 1: Setting Yourself Up For Success

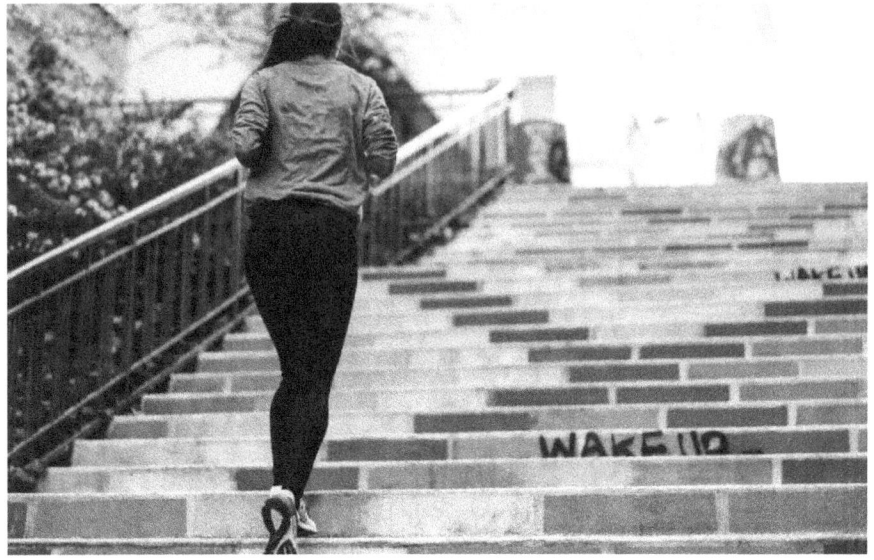

Photo by Ev on Unsplash

How Your Diet Affects Your Results

Exercise and diet are equally important factors to building muscle and losing fat. It is generally touted that diet may even play a larger role in the outcome of your fitness. If you are working out hard and not seeing results, make sure that the things you are eating are unprocessed and have high nutrient values—more specifically, work with a nutritionist to find the macronutrient intake levels that are right for the goal you are trying to reach.

Warm Up Before Working Out

To avoid injury, we should take some time before starting our workout to warm up all of our muscle groups. It is generally accepted that warming up before a workout will lead to better performance results and decrease the chance of injuring yourself. Don't forget to stretch after you're done, too! Warming up and cooling down should take no less than 5 minutes, but no more than 15-20 minutes. We don't want all your time spent prepping for your workout or stretching afterward, but they are important components that ensure your body's continued functionality.

Example Warm Up Workouts:

Complete these exercises for 5-10 minutes

1. Jog, row, or ride a bike at a slow-medium pace
2. Jump rope
3. High knees or butt kicks
4. Walk-out planks
5. Jumping jacks

Important Areas to Stretch:

Areas are followed by examples

1. Arms: arm circles
2. Legs: walking lunges
3. Glutes: glute bridge
4. Calves: wall lean
5. Back: leg pull

When warming up, we want our heart rate to increase, so make sure that while you are completing these exercises, you are adequately exerting yourself. We want our body to be ready for the more intense activity we are about to take part in. An increase in blood flow, an increase in body temperature, and an increase in breathing rate all build slowly through warming up in preparation. If you need to ask yourself if you are working out vigorously enough, a good test to check is to see if you would be able to keep a conversation going with your friend. If you are working out hard enough, you really shouldn't be able to keep a conversation going.

Who These Workouts Are Best-Suited For

Bodyweight Workouts are best-suited for those who cannot afford a gym membership, don't enjoy the gym atmosphere, or for those who feel like they are too large to jump right into fast-paced routines. Memberships can be expensive depending on where you go, and we don't all have enough money to afford one at certain points in our lives. Many people—women, in particular—feel uncomfortable at the gym or are intimidated by the size of the facility and the variety of equipment. Bodyweight Workouts can be modified for someone of any shape and size and can be completed in the privacy of your own home if you are self-conscious by working out in public.

Benefits of Bodyweight Workouts

These workouts allow you to build muscle, gain strength, and increase your stamina by using nothing other than your body. Able to be completed anywhere and with no equipment, Bodyweight Workouts are fast and effective. The Huffington Post contributor Dave Smith lists the numerous benefits of Bodyweight Workouts:

1. <u>They are efficient</u>: "Research suggests high-output, bodyweight-based exercises such as plyometrics yield awesome fitness gains in very short workout durations. Since there's no equipment involved, bodyweight workouts make it easy to transition quickly from one exercise to the next. Shorter rest times mean it's easy to boost heart rate and burn some serious calories quickly."

2. <u>There's something for everyone</u>: "Bodyweight exercises are a great choice because they're easily modified to challenge any fitness level. Adding extra repetitions, performing the exercises faster or super-slow, and perfecting form are a few ways to make even the simplest exercise more challenging. And progress is easy to measure since bodyweight exercises offer endless ways to do a little more in each workout."

3. <u>They can improve core strength</u>: "The 'core' is not just the abs. At least 29 muscles make up our core. Many bodyweight movements can be used to engage all of them. These will improve core strength, resulting in better posture and improved athletic performance."

4. <u>Workouts are convenient</u>: "Ask someone why they don't exercise. Chances are they'll answer they have 'no time' or that it's an 'inconvenience.' These common obstacles are eliminated by

bodyweight exercises because they allow anyone to squeeze in workouts any time, anywhere. It can be a stress reliever for those who work at home, or it can be a great hotel room workout for people on the road. With bodyweight workouts, 'no time' becomes no excuse."

5. <u>Workouts can be fun and easily mixed up for variety:</u> "It can be easy to get stuck in a workout rut of bench presses, lat pull-downs, and biceps curls. That's why bodyweight training can be so refreshing: There are countless exercise variations that can spice up any workout routine. Working with a variety of exercises not only relieves potential workout boredom, but it can also help break through exercise plateaus to spark further fitness progress."

6. <u>They can provide quick results</u>: "Bodyweight exercises get results partly because they often involve compound movements. Compound exercises such as push-ups, lunges, and chin-ups have been shown to be extremely effective for strength gains and performance improvements."

Creating a Workout Environment

Since these workouts can be complete at home, making sure you have available space to complete exercises is imperative for success. All you really need is a space large enough to spread out a little bit—let's say for example, to complete 10 lunges in a row. While you do not need any equipment, it may be nice to have a yoga mat if you have hard floors like wood or linoleum.

Some prefer a quiet environment to work out or to use a music player to help them focus during their workout. Do whatever puts you in the zone to complete your routine. The point is to try to minimize the space of distractions so you can put in the work to meet your goals.

Summary and Key Points

- Bodyweight Workouts are easy, fast, and are extremely effective for beginners and more seasoned exercisers!
- You can't expect the most comprehensive results without also ensuring your diet falls in line with the changes you want to see on your body!
- Designate a space to complete your workouts in, whether that be your living room or backyard patio.
- Design your space to allow for workout completion depending on space needs and create motivational vibes in the area for inspiration.

Chapter 2: Types of Bodyweight Workouts

Bodyweight workouts can be focused on targeting a specific group of muscles. This chapter will outline bodyweight exercises that target the following areas: arms, legs, chest, back, butt, and abs.

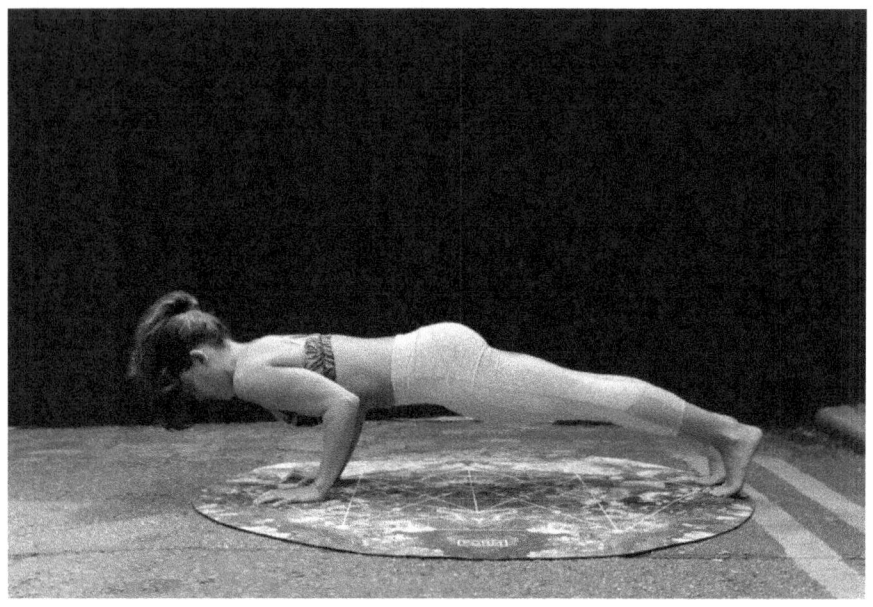

Photo by Form on Unsplash

We all have what we call 'problem areas,' and strength training can be the best and fastest way to target those areas on our bodies that we want to be more toned. Bodyweight Workouts use our own weight to create resistance so we can work on building up muscle on whichever body parts need our attention. Here are some examples of workouts from the before-named areas:

Focus: Arms

- **Tricep Dips**
    - This move helps build up your pectorals, triceps, forearms, and shoulder muscles. Push your chest out and using your arms, lower your body until your elbows are at 90 degrees. Push back up. Keep your head and chin up during the process.

- **Crab Walk**
    - Get down into a crab position: hands and feet in line with each other and flat on the ground with your chest facing up not down, knees bent, and hips held several inches off the ground. Walk several spaces forward, and then several spaces back.

    - Narrowing your hand placement while completing pushups will engage your core while toning your triceps, pectorals, and shoulders. Start in a pushup position, but instead of your hands lining up with your shoulders, move them in slightly on both sides. Lower your body down, holding yourself up, then push back into the starting position.

Focus: Legs

- **Wall Sit**

- Set your back up against a stable wall until your knees form a 90-degree angle with the wall. Your head, shoulders, and upper back should be lying flat against the wall, with your weight evenly distributed between both feet.

- **Jump Squat**
  - Standing straight up, keep your arms down by your sides. Squat down normally until your upper thighs are as close to parallel with the floor as they can be. Pressing off with your feet, jump straight up into the air, and as you touch down, go back into the squatting position and start again.

- **Lunges**
  - Starting in a standing position, head and chin up, eyes forward, take a step forward with one leg ensuring your knee is above your ankle. You don't want your other knee to touch the ground. Push back up into standing position and step forward with your opposite leg.

Focus: Chest

- **Incline Pushups**
  - This form is a great modification for those who may just be beginning and are struggling to do a basic pushup. Find some kind of incline in your workout area: a desk,

wall, chair, etc. and stand facing the incline with your feet shoulder width apart and feet 1-2 feet back from the wall. Place your hands on either side of the incline and place them slightly wider than your shoulders. Slowly bend the elbows and lower your body toward the incline, pause and push back up—try not to lock your elbows.

- **Traditional Plank**
  - Start off in a pushup position. Instead of lowering yourself and pushing yourself back up, you intend to hold your body in that position. Do not bend your elbows and make sure your feet are not wider than your shoulders. Hold this pose for 10 seconds to begin, and as you begin to master this exercise, work your way up to 30 seconds, 1 minute, etc.

- **Burpees**
  - This move combines several moves into one and can be a killer workout for beginners. Standing straight up, bend down in a position with your hands on the floor supporting your body. Kick back both feet until you are in a plank/pushup position. Quickly jump back on your feet and spring up, raising your hands to the sky. After lowering your arms, start again by bending back down.

Focus: Back

- **Reverse Snow Angel**

- o Instead of lying on your back like you were about to make a snow angel, flip over and lay face down on the ground. Raise your arms and shoulders off the ground slightly, about two inches, and bring your hands down from your sides up past your head. (If you were standing not laying down you would be raising and lowering your arms in an up and down wing-flapping motion.)

- **Superman**
    - o Lie face down on the ground with your toes pointing down under your body. Reach your arms out straight to your sides, and raise both your arms and feet in the air while making sure your torso maintains contact with the ground.

- **Good Mornings aka Hip Hinges**
    - o Standing up straight with your hands on your hips and your feet shoulder-width apart, bend forward at your waist until your back is parallel to the ground. Engage your core and bring your torso back up in a straight position. It is important to keep your neck in line with your spine while doing this exercise.

Focus: Butt

- **Fire Hydrants**

- ○ Start in a modified pushup position—the standard pushup position but with knees and hands on the ground instead of feet and hands on the ground. Raise one leg off the ground with your knee bent at a 90-degree angle. This move can also be completed with a straight leg for similar results. If you need inspiration, you want to look like a dog who is just about the use a fire hydrant!

- **Leg Kickbacks**
  - ○ Again, start in a modified pushup position. Try to align your shoulders with your knees. Kick one leg back behind you. Make sure you feel the movement in your hips and glutes, not your lower back. Bring your leg back down and switch sides.

- **Glute Bridges**
  - ○ Lay on the ground, flat on your back with your hands by your sides. Place your feet flat on the floor shoulder-width apart. Use your upper back, upper arms, and core to raise your hips up off the ground toward the sky while keeping your feet and arms on the ground. Slowly lower your hips until they are resting back on the ground.

Focus: Abs

- **Side Planks**

- Lie down on your side on the floor, and place one elbow underneath you so that you are forming a plank on one side. Keeping your elbow underneath your shoulder, push your lower torso up off of the ground so that the only things touching the ground are your right forearm and the side of your right foot or your left forearm and the side of your left foot. Hold the position for ten seconds, release, and then resume the position.

- **Flutter Kicks**
  - Lie on your back on the floor with your arms down by your sides and your heels flat on the ground. Lift your heels about 6 inches off the ground, and quickly kick your legs up and down. It is easier to complete 10 kicks, rest for 20 seconds, then do another 10 kicks because of how short and quick the kicks are.

- **V-Sit Crunch**
  - Lay flat on your back on the ground with your arms laying above your head. Lift up your legs like you are about to attempt a crunch, but bring your arms up toward your legs at the same time, creating a 'V.' Lower your arms and legs back into the starting position lying down.

Summary and Key Points

- There are many more exercises within each focus category. The ones listed in this book are just suggestions to get you started.
- If you are confused about how to complete an exercise, YouTube has an excellent variety of step-by-step videos.
- It's a great idea to track your repetitions (reps), so you know you started being able to do 10 pushups and now doing 25!

Chapter 3: Planning a Workout Routine That Works For You

Bodyweight workouts are perfect because it can be completed with only some space and your body: no gym or equipment required! An even better bonus to these exercises is that they are so simple to do that they are easily combined to reap even more benefits in the same amount of time.

What to Include In Your Plan

Important aspects of a workout routine include duration, frequency, intensity, and consistency. The Mayo Clinic suggests adults get in about 150 minutes of moderate exercise a week, or 75 minutes of vigorous activity and at least 2 days of strength training: "Moderate aerobic exercise includes activities such as brisk walking, swimming, and mowing the lawn. Vigorous aerobic exercise includes activities such as running and aerobic dancing. Strength training can include the use of weight machines, your own body weight, resistance tubing, resistance paddles in the water, or activities such as rock climbing."

To break this down for you, you should look at workouts with moderate intensity for 3 days a week for 50 minutes each, or 5 days a week for 30 minutes each. It's up to you to decide when you want to schedule your workouts throughout the week, but making sure you start your Mondays with a workout is always a great way to set up your week for success!

How to Stay Dedicated When Your Resolve Falters

A LifeHacker article written by Alan Henry has some great tips on how to motivate yourself to start your routine and how to stick with your routine. Without consistency, you will never see or keep results!

1. Stop Making Excuses

   - Don't be too hard on yourself, we all make mistakes and expect too much from ourselves. Know that failures are an expected part of the journey.

   - We all have to start from somewhere—doing something, no matter how small, is better than doing nothing at all!

2. Understand Your Habits

   - "Most people fail in fitness because they never enter a self-sustaining positive feedback loop. To be successful at fitness, it needs to be in the same category of the brain as sleeping, eating, and sex." The key is to find a routine replacement that works for you and gets results for the energy you put into building it into your habits."

   - Starting from zero can cause people to want to give up: "Oftentimes, people are actually lazy because they're out of shape and don't exercise!" It's quite easy for a fit person to tell someone who's having a tough time that they're just lazy, but the reality is that running a mile is much easier for someone who does five every day compared to someone who's been sitting on the couch for most of his life."

3. Find Your "Secret Sauce"
    - "Minimizing and oversimplifying the challenge doesn't help, and while hearing what worked for others can help you figure out things to try, it's almost never going to be exactly what works for you. Look for your own combination of tools, tips, techniques, and advice that will support you and your health and fitness goals."

4. Be Engaged and Stick to Your Plan
    - "Set the bar low and start small. If you're having trouble with working out every day, start with twice or once a week. Whatever it is, start with something you can *definitely* do effortlessly. This is where suggestions like parking on the far end of the lot and taking the stairs come into play."

    - "Whatever you do, make it fun. Whatever you do, enjoy it. Choose something rewarding enough to make you feel good about doing it. If you're having a good time, mistakes feel like learning experiences and challenges to be overcome, not throw-up-your-hands-and-give-up moments."

5. Track Your Victories With Technology
   - "Technology can be a huge benefit to help you see your progress in a way that looking in the mirror won't show you. The goal is to keep that track record, whether it's on a calendar, in an app, or on a website, going unbroken as long as possible. Just remember, quantifying your efforts is just a method to get feedback and track your progress. Your tech should be a means to build better habits, not the habit in itself."

Another great way to keep yourself accountable is by enlisting a friend to work out with you. Even if you don't have the same fitness goals or you don't want to be distracted while you are trying to work out, having someone to be accountable to can really push us to meet our goals. Whether that's a text or a phone call on days you know your friend should be working out, that small reminder may be enough to get them going.

Sample 7-day Routine

After deciding how many days and for how long each day you want to work out, the next step is planning what exercises you will complete in each session. It's not generally recommended that you focus on the same muscle groups two days in a row, although every other day is absolutely fine!

Sunday: Arms

15 pushups x3

15 tricep dips x3

15 lay down pushup x3

15 walkouts x3

Monday: Legs

15 jump squats x3

16 X jumps x3

15 lunges x3

24 high knees x3

10 burpees x3

Tuesday: Rest!

Wednesday: Chest

10 second plank x3

15 decline pushups x3

15 mountain climbers x3

15 burpees x3

Thursday: Abs

    15 straight leg sit ups x3

    20 ab bikes x3

    15 straight leg raises x3

    20 side twists

Friday: Rest!

Saturday: Back

    15 bridges x3

    15 back extensions x3

    15 opposite arm/leg raises x3

    15 bridges x3

Try to complete all four workouts on each day as fast as you can while resting for up to 30 seconds between each move. If you want to up the intensity, slowly increase the repetitions—a good interval is an increase of 5. Another way to make the workout more intense is to complete the workout as a circuit. If you complete a day's workouts as a circuit, ignore the "repeat 3 times." Instead, you would complete, for example, 15 straight leg sit-ups, 20 ab bikes, 15 straight leg raises, and 20 side twists. Rest for 30 seconds! Repeat starting with 15 straight leg sit-ups. Try to not rest for more than 30 seconds. If you need to when you're just beginning, that's completely okay! Complete one circuit and begin working on adding additional circuits to your workouts.

If you already have a workout routine that you regularly complete, try adding in certain strength training exercises between your cardio workout. Again, slowly build up your repetitions but starting small.

Summary and Key Points

- Plan your workouts into your day with your planner or calendar system. Start small and build your way up to working out 3, 4, or 5 days a week!
- Switch up the muscle groups you focus on to make sure that you see full body results.
- The recommended workouts are only a very small example of workouts within each category to get you started. Research muscle groups you want to target and incorporate those goals into your workout plan.

Chapter 4: How to Make the Most Out of Your Bodyweight Workouts

As touched on in the last chapter regarding circuit workouts, High-Intensity Interval Training is a great way to target multiple muscle groups in one workout and burn more calories. We will also touch on tools that can be used to track your workouts and your progress, as well as an important aspect of ending your workout that is sometimes forgotten but still important: stretching!

High-Intensity Interval Training

According to Bodybuilding.com, "these different body compositions point to the fact that not all cardio is created equal, which is why it's important to choose a form of cardio that meets your goals. A recent study compared participants who did steady-state cardio for 30 minutes three times a week to those who did 20 minutes of high-intensity interval training (HIIT) three times per week. Both groups showed similar weight loss, but the HIIT group showed a 2 percent loss in body fat while the steady-state group lost only 0.3 percent. The HIIT group also gained nearly two pounds of muscle, while the steady-state group lost almost a pound."

Progress Can Be Small, But Any Progress is Significant

Tracking your gains is an important part of using body weight workouts. Some people prefer creating their own systems in a notebook or journal, others use electronic devices, and the rest of us prefer to use visual progress indicators.

Writing down when you completed a workout, what exercises you completed, and how many repetitions you completed is a great reminder of your goals and how far you've come on the journey to reach them. Before your next workout, refer back to your last logged workout and see what adjustments you need to make to your workout today to help you be successful.

Technology Can Help Us Keep More Accurate Records

Using a tracking device like a Fitbit watch, hybrid smartwatch, iPhone, or smart shoes, you can track calories burned, distance moved, heart rate, and then have them saved somewhere digitally instead of in a hard copy paper form.

Stretching for Injury Prevention Should Be a Priority

Warming up and then stretching after a workout is an important way to help prevent injuries. Stretch out your arms, legs, back, and any other areas that feel tight.

Key Summary Points

- HIIT workouts are a great way to combine targeting different muscle groups in one workout instead of many.

- Tracking your gains in whichever fashion makes you the most comfortable and that you find the most motivating is highly encouraged!

Taking 5-15 minutes to stretch after a workout will ease soreness for your workouts in the following days, and will help prevent your muscles from getting injured.

Conclusion

Back pain is experienced by a large portion of our society, and many go undiagnosed and without help for many years. You may feel exhausted, trying several methods to alleviate your back, neck, and shoulder pain and feel as though you have no hope at feeling better. The truth is, there are many incredible alternative solutions that can help you feel much better from your back, neck, or shoulder pain.

Being open to trying new things could be the difference between having pain, or living pain-free. This book is full of methods that can help eliminate your pain and keep you healthy and with a higher quality of life for much longer. Remember, if you are experiencing a medical emergency or your back pain is a result of something medical, you should always use alternative therapies with caution and as a part of your regular healing routine. They are an important addition, but should not always be considered the sole solution in every circumstance. You must consider your unique health and wellness and choose the best course of action that will not interfere with your overall wellbeing.

www.ingramcontent.com/pod-product-compliance
Lightning Source LLC
LaVergne TN
LVHW020447070526
838199LV00063B/4875